Ms. Dee's Journey:

Breast Cancer

Betty Mattin

Ms. Dee's Journey: Breast Cancer

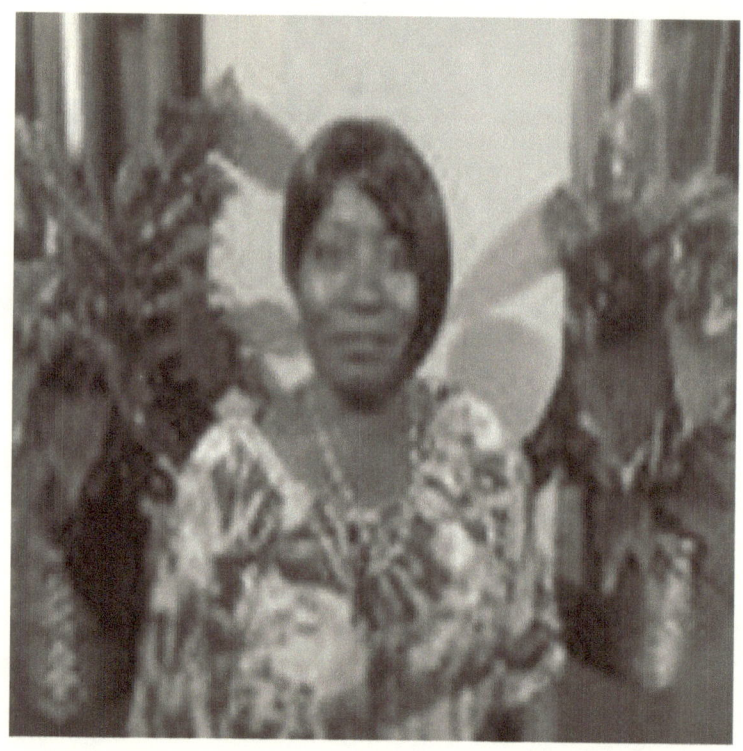

"He took up our infirmities and carried our diseases."
Matthew 8:17

Table of Contents

Acknowledgments

Special thanks to Columbus Regional, Columbus Hospice, John Amos Cancer Center, Cheryl Carden Breast Cancer Foundation, Theresa Osborne, Dr. Motiwalla and his staff, Dr. Hudson and others who helped Ms. Dee during her journey. May God keep and bless you all.

Cancer

You touch the bodies of the living

And mark them for dead

A plague of their own flesh

Rampant, raging, you spread.

Cruel monster, slithering

Through vessels, unknown

Multiplying, dividing

You plunder, you grow

You ravage and destroy

Rot the body like wood

No care for the innocent

No mercy for the good.

Blood, swelling, horror

When, at last, you are found

We fight for the victim

To which you are bound

We poison you, poison

Hack, gauge you out

Burn you, hot waves

Just kill you somehow

Internal struggles, a war

That won't make the news

Sometimes we win

And sometimes

We lose.

-by Amina Bhatti

(www.heartfulwhispers.blogspot.com)

Ms. Dee's Journey

"The Lord Is My Shepherd, and I Shall Not Want"
(Psalm:23)

E ven through her pain and troubles, Ms. Dee touched many people's lives. Her inspiration, strength, love for God and willingness to help others will live on within this book. People need to realize and understand that, no matter what you are going through, "God is still in control;" that was her favorite saying. People come into our lives for a reason and a season. When they both have served their purpose, God removes them from our midst. She entered into many people's lives for a season and then God said, "My child, it's time for you to depart their lives."

Others were for a reason and her wish was that those individuals learn something from her. If Ms. Dee was in your life for either a season or reason, then she left a great impact on your life. Just remember the things that she said to you. It may have been scripture, a story she shared with you or just her ear when you needed someone to listen. She may not be here physically, but she is always here spiritually and will be missed.

This book is here to guide and inspire anyone who is going through cancer. To let you know that, no matter what you are going through, God will bring you through it. God can do any and everything but fail you. The will of God is always going to overrule the will that we have for our loved ones. God knows what is best for us. When he does something in our lives, it's for a reason, and the reason is for us to learn a lesson from it. Take life by the horns and enjoy it while you can. Stop dwelling on your illness because that is when the illness will take control. You take control over the illness. I hope something been said that will carry you through your illness and everyday life.

Remember these words from Ms. Dee: "Prayer is the key and faith unlock the door." She stood on these words in her everyday walk with Jesus and knew they would bring her through.

Ms. Dee's Journey Begins:

Cast All Your Cares on Jesus

Psalm 56:3 "but when I am afraid, I will put my trust in you"

My journey began as a breast cancer victim. "The Lord is My Shephard ... I Shall Not Want" (November 9,2009).

I had a meeting at Department Family Assistance Child Services (DFACS) to get some medical assistance. I was afraid I would not get it but God is always on-time. (October 26, 2009)

Patiently waiting for answers. In the meantime, my breast is on fire. (October 27, 2009)

Still waiting. I made an appointment with Dr. Motiwalla. Appointment on October 29,2009. (October 28,2009)

Went to see Dr. Motiwalla. He was upset about the way my breast looked. He knew what my odds were, but was afraid to tell me, so he immediately sent me to the breast cancer center for a biopsy the next day. He had a concerned look on his face. Yes, I was afraid of the outcome. (October 29, 2009)

I went for the biopsy. At this point, I knew my fate (life) was completely in God's hands. He's not leaving me. (October 30,2009)

Praying for my health, not stressing. (October31 - November 3,2009)

I found out I had breast cancer. Delisa and Keyla were with me. For some reason, I was already in acceptance of what God had planned for me. I knew he would not put more on me than I could handle. I am his child and he only want the best for me. I know God loves me and that's all that matters. Dr. Motiwalla got right on the situation. I was ready to begin my journey. 1st path report IBC. (November 4, 2009)

I'm just praying. (November 5,2009)

The devil put plenty of bad thoughts in my mind. I refuse to give in because I knew, "God is in control." I just needed to keep my faith and listen to God. He has a special job for me while I am on my breast cancer journey. (November 6,2009)

CANCER IS SO LIMITED

It cannot cripple LOVE.
It cannot shatter HOPE.
It cannot corrode FAITH.
It cannot destroy CONFIDENCE.
It cannot kill FRIENDSHIP.
It cannot shout out MEMORIES.
It cannot silence COURAGE.
It cannot invade the SOUL.
It cannot destroy PEACE.
It cannot quench the SPIRIT.
It cannot lessen the
POWER OF THE RESURRECTION.
IT CANNOT STEAL ETERNAL LIFE.
Our greatest enemy is not the disease, but despair.
Keep trusting God's love so that your spirit will remain strong.
If cancer has invaded your life, refuse to let it touch your
SPIRIT.
Your body can be severely afflicted, and you can have great
struggle,
but if you keep trusting in God's love,
Your SPIRIT will remain strong!

(Unknown author)

Psalm 30:5: Weeping may endure for a night but joy cometh in the morning

Hard to even celebrate CJ's (first-born grandson) 6th birthday. Constantly thinking about the future outcome for my children. Debating about talking to Dr. Chambers about the cabbage leaf deal. (November 7-8, 2009)

Went to see Dr. Smith, a breast surgeon. He didn't cut any corners; he told me that my breast had to be cut off, then I said, "Well, just take both of them." I was startled about my illness; however, it is what it is. Aunt Dot was with me. She made me feel so comfortable. I remember being at the Breast Center alone and God appeared to me and said, "I've never left you before, and I'm here for you and will always be here." I never really believed in the spirit speaking to anyone like this until now. It's real. I know it is. I must be strong for my children. I was in terrible pain all the time. (November 7-8, 2009)

I had my chemo port put in. My oncologist was Dr. Palmer at the Amos. S-28 was my number while I was at the Medical Center. At this point, Delisa, Keyla and my family are my greatest supporters. Head thinks I'm contagious, that is okay. God is going to see me through this. 2nd diagnosis (infiltration grade 2 apocrine mammary carcinoma) I feared nothing. I am human, so my flesh does get weak. God, please give me the strength to get through your plan. (November 10, 2009)

Sore, but living. I wanted to give my children much love as possible. I want Candy to get her children back. I believe she can do it. God please help me to help her. (November 11,2009)

Ahmani's pegs are showing. I am glad to have had the opportunity to see them first. She's so cute. (November 19,2009)

Eco wasn't good...Got to keep moving.... (November. 20,2009)

I will start my first 3 chemo tabs. (November 22,2009)

Went to Chemo class. Began chemo. I was told my hair would come out, as well as the hair on my body. My family is here for the holidays. Aunt Dot, Delisa, Candy and Keyla went to chemo with me. I was happy to have them there with me. (November 23,2009)

John 15:11 "These things I have spoken to you that my joy may remain in you and that your joy may be full"

I enjoyed my family despite my illness. I was hurting but I didn't tell them. (November 24-27, 2009)

These days were fair. I worked that Monday. I must keep going no matter what; I like my own money. (November 28-30, 2009)

Prepared for PET. I prayed that no other cancer would be found anywhere else on my body. This body belongs to GOD! (December 1, 2009)

PET was EXCELLENT! Thank you! For no man could do what God does, He's in control! Romans 8:38,39: For I am persuaded beyond doubt (am sure) that neither death, nor life, nor angels, nor principalities, nor things and threatening, nor things to come, nor power, nor height, nor depth, nor anything else in all creation will be able to separate us from the love of God, which is in Christ Jesus our Lord." (December 2, 2009)

I went to work.... (December. 3, 2009)

Uncle Jim went to the hospital. He wasn't doing good. (December 4,2009)

Uncle Jim died in Tifton General Hospital. I knew his illness but will never tell. He's resting in peace with no pain. God called home.... (December 5, 2009)

I cut my hair off due to it coming out. I don't look bad. I am a bald DIVA! Keyla took pictures of me showing off my beauty. (December, 2009)

Nay was here with us for Christmas. I wanted my twins' first Christmas to be the best. I literally had to beg Head to buy them something but he said they were too little. (December 2009)

VICTORIOUS! I thank God each day! It wasn't a cakewalk but I am here. My truck was needing some work. Nobody helped me with the maintenance on it, therefore I am the chief in the front seat. God made it possible for me to buy my truck and I am going to enjoy it.

Received truck back from Ms. Miles. (January 2010)

They changed my chemo medication due to abnormal reading. The rest of the month was fair. I started the death pill, Xeloda. I begin my 4th round of chemo and it has been going well. (January 18, 2010)

I am Thankful: God's Abundant Blessings

Psalm 120:1 "In my distress I cried unto the Lord and he heard me."

I would like to thank God for my adopted daughter, Shawnise, because she was there with me every step of the way. She came up to the breast cancer unit with me when I took my chemo treatments. Shawinse would even miss days from school in order to be there for me when I was taking chemo. She is such an inspiration for me. With Shawnise, you would never know what she was up to. She always had a ram in the bush. All of my adopted children were there for me and they treated me like a queen. I knew that I did not run this race in vain. I just hope that my friends, family and others learned something from my journey.

I began to get sick....

February 2010 was the last entry into Ms. Dee's journey in her own words. As the months went by, she became sicker and sicker, but no matter what, she kept pressing on for herself and for her family. She knew what the will of God would do for her and how it would lead her. She knew that God said, by his strife we are already healed. Nothing could separate her from the love and belief in Jesus Christ. I can remember the day she accepted Christ and was baptized. It was an amazing day to see my beloved friend give God her heart and the pastor her hand.

On December 19, 2010, my beloved friend crossed over into eternal life. I know my beloved friend is in heaven, PAIN FREE, walking tall in her new body.

Ms. Dee's Favorite Scriptures That Kept Her During her Time of Need

Jeremiah 29:12: "Then you will call upon me and go and pray to me, and I will listen to you.

Romans 8-18: My pain will not be wasted

For I consider that the sufferings of this

present time (this present life)

are not worth being compared with the

glory that is about be revealed to us

and for us and conferred on us!

1. Peter 1:6,7

"Humble yourselves, therefore, under God's mighty hand, that he may lift you up in due time. Cast all your anxiety on him because he cares for you."

2. John 16:33

"I have told you these things so that, in me, you may have peace. In this world, you will have trouble. But take heart! I have overcome the world."

3. Ephesians 4:26, 27

"In your anger do not sin" [a]: Do not let the sun go down while you are still angry; 27. and do not give the devil a foothold.

4. James 1:6

But when he asks, he must believe and not doubt, because he who doubts is like a wave of the sea, blown and tossed by the wind.

5. Isaiah 41:10

So do not fear, for I am with you; do not be dismayed, for I am your God. I will strengthen you and help you; I will upload you with my righteous right hand.

6. 2 Timothy 1:12

I know whom I have believed and am convinced that he is able to guard what I have entrusted to him for that day.

7. Romans 8:15

You did not receive a spirit that makes you a slave again to fear, but you received the Spirit of sonship. And by him, we cry, "Abba, Father."

8. Psalm 23:3-4

He restores my soul. He guides me in paths of righteousness for his name's sake. Even though I walk through the valley of the shadow of death, I will fear no evil, for you are with me; your rod and your staff, they comfort me.

Now it's time for you to start your journey. Writing is a very therapeutic technique that will help you gather your thoughts and, maybe one day, help someone. God gives us a test so that we might give a testimony. People can only believe and press on in life if they hear the great miracles God has already performed. Let your journey be a testimony to others.

On the next pages, you will write your name on the blank line and start your journey. I wish you well in your journey and may God bless you.

Ms. Dee's sister in Christ,

Betty Martin-Woods.

You are truly missed, my beloved sister.

"As the Winds of Time Blow" - Anonymous

As the winds of time blow softly

and whisper so you can hear,

I really love and miss you, nan,

and wish you were still here.

Betty Mattin

_____Journey Begin On_____

_____Journey Begin On_____

_____Journey Begin On_____

_____Journey Begin On_____

Betty Mattin

_____Journey Begin On_____

Comforting Quotes from Other Cancer Patients

"If children have the ability to ignore all odds and percentages, then maybe we can all learn from them. When you think about it, what other choice is there but to hope? We have two options, medically and emotionally: give up, or fight like hell."
-Lance Armstrong

"Cancer is a word, not a sentence."
John Diamond

"Courage is being afraid but going on anyhow."
Dan Rather

"The only courage that matters is the kind that gets you from one moment to the next."
Mignon McLaughlin

"Courage is fear that has said its prayers."
Dorothy Bernard

"The human spirit is stronger than anything that can happen to it."
C.C. Scott

"Physical strength is measured by what we can carry; spiritual by what we can bear."
Author Unknown

"Toughness is in the soul and spirit, not in muscles."
Alex Karras

"Adversity is like a strong wind. It tears away from us all but the things that cannot be torn, so that we see ourselves as we really are."
Arthur Golden

"Oh, my friend, it's not what they take away from you that counts—it's what you do with what you have left."
Hubert Humphrey

"If you're going through hell, keep going."
Winston Churchill

"We acquire the strength we have overcome."
Ralph Waldo Emerson

"Hope is that thing with feathers that perches in the soul and sings the tune without the words and never stops ... at all."
Emily Dickinson

"Time is shortening. But every day that I challenge this cancer and survive is a victory for me."
Ingrid Bergman

"I don't think of all the misery but of the beauty that still remains."
Anne Frank

"Never, never, never give up."
Winston Churchill

"Do not be afraid of tomorrow, for God is already there."
Author Unknown

"You gain strength, courage and confidence by every experience in which you really stop to look fear in the face."
Eleanor Roosevelt

"You never know how strong you are until being strong is the only choice you have."
Cayla Mills

_____Journey Begin On_____

_____Journey Begin On_____

Betty Mattin

_____Journey Begin On_____

_____Journey Begin On_____

_____Journey Begin On_____

_____Journey Begin On_____

"The Cancer Devil" by Patty Ritter

Copywritten@ 2005","Patty Ritter Virginia Beach, Virginia

The Cancer Devil came to me

And whispered thoughtless pain

He chooses to take my little girl into the cancer rain.

I begged him to go away and leave us all alone

Yet, He choose to stay, instead, to prepare her for his home.

Yet, we stood strong despite the pain

We still live on despite the rain,

When the road of Life comes back,

We'll send the Cancer Devil to his Final Rest.

_____Journey Begin On_____

Betty Mattin

_____Journey Begin On_____

"Humble Cry" by Sherry Maxwell

Cure, dear Christ, the cancer

That seeps within my soul

You, Lord, are the answer

You can make me whole

Bring me, Lord, your mercy

And your loving grace

Show me what I'd dare seek

Turn to me your face

Miraculous Redeemer

Gentle Shepherd King

Light of heaven, bring near

Praises now I sing

Lord of all creation

Ruler of the sky

Know my adoration

Hear my humble cry.

_____Journey Begin On_____

_____Journey Begin On_____

Words from Ms. Dee

PRAYER IS THE KEY; faith keeps the door open. Keeping God FIRST is a must. God's LOVE is the greatest love ever. Live every day to the minute as if it is your LAST.

To my family, I have accepted what God has for me. He used me for a reason which was not for me to understand but for you all to learn from. I love you all and I am in my new spiritual body, PAIN FREE. I will be waiting on you all, so get your life right so we can see each other again. Be courageous and encourage each other.

She said, I am a beautiful "Bald Diva"

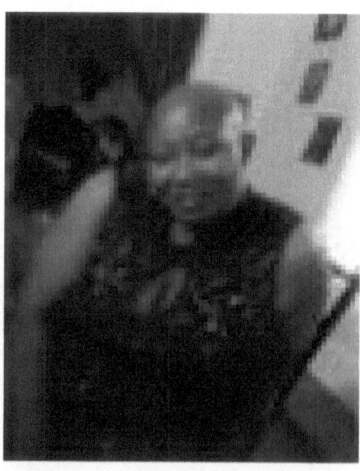

"In support" by Bernie D, PEI, CANADA

In support, I shaved my head and changed my look.

Just one small comment in life's great book.

I'm here for you, is all I mean.

To add strength and hope to all you dream.

Side by side, we will win this fight

Day by day and night by night.

No more dodging that double-edged knife.

We will be champions of this game called life.

Ms. Darlene Cooks-Sheffield, 36, blossomed on May 27, 1974 in Cordele, Georgia and resided in Columbus Georgia. She was called home on December 19, 2010 at Columbus Hospice in Columbus, Georgia.

Betty Mattin

_____Journey Begin On_____

_____Journey Begin On_____

_____Journey Begin On_____

_____Journey Begin On_____

Betty Mattin

_____Journey Begin On_____

_____Journey Begin On_____

Betty Mattin

_____Journey Begin On_____

_____Journey Begin On_____

Betty Mattin

_____Journey Begin On_____

_____Journey Begin On_____

"The Trail of Healing"

Left prints on the sand grains
Wind has erased once used to be a trail
Illness strays our life imprints
"Lord"- we are on weakness stand - enlighten us with hints
Inspire our soul towards the trail of healing
There comes a finding
We urge to be awakened from the frightening trance
Truth is, the spinning fate changes our journey in a glance
It's beyond the terrain chase searching for trace
The will glints from within
Faith, support—the need to believe in
The fight shall never end

By Nasra Al Adawi.

"TODAY IS A GIFT"

by LASZLO KOTRO-KOSZTANDI

Many people will walk in and out of your life,
But only true friends will leave footprints on your heart.
To handle yourself, use your head;
To handle others, use your heart.
Anger is only one letter short of danger.
If someone betrays you twice, it is your fault.
Great minds discuss events;
Small minds discuss people.
He who loses money, loses much;
He who loses a friend, loses much more;
He who loses faith, loses all.
Beautiful old people are works of art.
Learn from the mistakes of others.
You can't live long enough to make them all yourself.
Friends, you and me ... You brought another friend ... and we started our
group ... our circle of friends ... and like a circle ... There is no
beginning or end ... Yesterday is history.
Tomorrow is a mystery. Today is a gift.